Protection Guide From Ticks

Learn how to identify, remove, and protect yourself from these dangerous bloodsuckers

Sandra Vogel

Copyright

Table of Content

Introduction

Ticks Are Becoming a Greater Threat

Ticks are more than just a bother. They are small spider-like insects that attach themselves quietly to people and animals. They are parasites that feed on blood and can spread many dangerous diseases. Their numbers have been growing over the past few years, and they are becoming more common. Ticks carry a number of diseases that can be very sick or even deadly, so this growing threat has big effects on public health.

Ticks come in more than 800 different types, and 84 of them have been found in the United States alone. The blacklegged tick, which is also called the deer tick, is the most well-known of these. Not only are these ticks famous for being able to feed on blood, but they also spread Lyme disease, which is one of the most common tick-borne diseases in the U.S. The lone star tick, the American dog tick, and the brown dog tick are some other popular ticks. Each of these ticks can spread its own set of diseases.

Ticks like places with lots of tall grass, dense plants, and leaf litter. Because of this, they are often found with people when they are hiking, camping, or farming outside. Their life cycle includes three stages: worm, nymph, and adult. At each stage, they require a blood meal to move to the next. Both male and female ticks feed on blood, but it is the female ticks that become engorged to the size of a pea after feeding, a sight that can be alarming when found on one's skin.

The diseases that ticks carry and transmit to humans and animals are a main concern. Lyme disease, caused by the bacterium *Borrelia burgdorferi*, is the most well-known tick-borne illness. It can lead to severe health problems if not treated quickly, including arthritis, neurological issues, and heart problems. The blacklegged tick is the main vector for this disease, and its nymphs, which are about the size of a poppy seed, are particularly adept at going unnoticed until they have fed sufficiently.

However, Lyme disease is not the only threat. The lone star tick, for instance, can spread ehrlichiosis and Southern tick-associated rash illness (STARI). More alarmingly, its bite can introduce a sugar molecule into the bloodstream that causes an allergy to red meat, a condition known as alpha-gal syndrome. This allergy can be severe, leading to anaphylactic reactions in some people. The American dog tick is known to spread Rocky Mountain spotted fever, a possibly fatal disease if not treated early.

The spread of ticks and the diseases they carry is exacerbated by climate change and growing urbanization. Warmer temperatures and milder winters contribute to the growth of tick habitats and extend their active seasons. Suburban development often puts humans into closer contact with tick habitats, increasing the chance of encounters.

Given the growing threat posed by ticks, knowing how to prevent tick bites and what to do if bitten is crucial. Preventative measures include using insect repellents containing DEET, picaridin, or oil of lemon eucalyptus, which are good against ticks. Wearing protective clothes, such as long sleeves and pants tucked into socks, can also help. Additionally, treating clothes and gear with permethrin, an insecticide that kills ticks on contact, is highly effective. After spending time outdoors, it is important to perform thorough tick checks on oneself, children, and pets, and to promptly remove any ticks found.

Removing a tick should be done carefully to reduce the risk of disease transmission. Using fine-tipped tweezers, grab the tick as close to the skin's surface as possible and pull upward with steady, even pressure. Avoid twisting or jerking the tick, as this can cause the mouthparts to break off and stay in the skin. Once removed, clean the bite area with soap and water or an antibiotic. It is recommended to save the tick in rubbing alcohol or hand sanitizer for identification in case of illness.

Chapter 1: Understanding What Ticks is

Little but dangerous, ticks are arachnids that are more than just a mere annoyance—they may seriously harm an animal's or human's health. It is essential to comprehend these animals in order to prevent and handle them effectively. We'll go over the common tick species in the US, their life cycle, and the distinctions between male and female ticks in this thorough review.

The United States' Tick Species

There are 84 known species of ticks in the United States, although only a small number are frequently linked to disease transmission through tick bites. The most famous of these are the brown dog tick, American dog itch, lone star tick, and blacklegged tick.

1. Ixodes scapularis, the blacklegged tick:

The blacklegged tick, also referred to as the deer tick, is the main carrier of the bacteria Borrelia burgdorferi, which causes Lyme disease. Northeastern and upper Midwestern regions of the United States are where it is most frequently found. In addition to Lyme disease, it can spread the Powassan virus, babesiosis, and anaplasmosis.

2. Amblyomma americanum, or Lone Star Tick:

The lone star tick, which is common in the southeast and eastern United States, can be identified by the white dot on the back of adult females. It is well known for dispersing Southern tick-associated rash sickness (STARI) and ehrlichiosis. Its bite can also result in red meat allergy by causing alpha-gal syndrome.

3. Dermacentor variabilis, the American dog tick:

Grassy and forested environments are frequent habitats for this tick, especially in the eastern United States and along the Pacific coast. Both tularemia and Rocky Mountain spotted fever (RMSF) can be spread by it.

4. Brown Dog Tick (Rhipicephalus sanguineus): This tick species is a major nuisance in dog kennels and households since it can live its whole life cycle indoors, in contrast to other tick species. It is a carrier of both babesiosis and canine ehrlichiosis.

A Tick's Life Cycle

The life cycle of a tick consists of four stages: egg, larva, nymph, and adult. Comprehending this cycle is crucial to understanding their behavior and the most effective ways to manage their populations.

1. Egg: In a protected area, a female tick lays hundreds of eggs to start the life cycle.

The six-legged larvae that emerge from these eggs are referred to as "seed ticks."

2. Larva: A tick's larval stage is its first period of activity. For their initial blood meal, these tiny larvae look for small hosts like rodents or birds. They leave their host after feeding and molt into eight-legged nymphs.

3. Nymph: Although comparatively smaller than larvae, nymphs are more significant and can be harder to find. For their blood meal, they hunt out larger hosts, including as people and dogs. Because nymphs can carry diseases from their earlier larval stage, this stage is particularly significant for the transmission of disease. They drop off and molt into adults after feeding.

4. Adult: For their last blood meal, adult ticks look for large hosts like humans, dogs, or deer. In particular, female ticks need a big blood meal in order to lay eggs. Female ticks lay eggs after feeding, restarting the cycle. Contrarily, male ticks frequently pass away following mating.

Ticks can live up to three years, and each stage of their life cycle can take many months to complete. They are hardy pests because of their extended lifespan and capacity for fasting.

Distinctions Between Ticks, Male and Female

Comprehending the distinctions between male and female ticks helps facilitate their identification and understanding as well as their functions in disease transmission and reproduction.

1. Size and Appearance: After feeding, female ticks tend to be larger than male ones. As they eat blood, females might become noticeably engorged, whilst males tend to be flatter and smaller. Additionally, there can be differences in coloration; males tend to be more uniform in their darker tones, while females may have unique markings, such as the white dot on female lone star ticks.

2. Feeding Behavior: Ticks feed on blood, but they do so in different ways for males and females. For the purpose of growing and laying eggs, females need a large blood meal. They swell dramatically when they become engorged. In contrast, males eat infrequently and are mainly concerned with locating partners. Males in many species may feed for limited periods of time and do not engorge like females do.

3. Reproductive Role: Finding and mating with female ticks is the main responsibility of male ticks. They have unique structures for mating, and they frequently stick with a female once they've found one. Throughout their lives, males may mate with several females. After mating and feasting, female

ticks concentrate on laying eggs. Because they are capable of laying hundreds of eggs, the tick population will always exist.

4. Disease Transmission: Ticks can carry diseases from male to female, but because females feed for longer periods of time, they are frequently more important carriers of disease. A tick is more likely to spread infections to its host the longer it is connected and feeding. Because of this, female ticks are especially significant when it comes to disease prevention and public health.

Disease and Ticks

Ticks are infamous for carrying a variety of diseases that can affect both humans and animals. When a tick feeds on an infected host and then feeds on another host, it spreads the infections it has acquired. This is how this transmission happens. The following are a few of the most prevalent tick-borne illnesses in the US:

1. Lyme Disease:

Mostly spread by the blacklegged tick, Lyme disease is caused by the bacteria *Borrelia burgdorferi*. Fever, headaches, exhaustion, and a rash resembling a bullseye are possible symptoms. Lyme disease can cause serious health complications, such as arthritis and neurological difficulties, if it is not treated.

2. Spotted fever of Rocky Mountains (RMSF):

Rickettsia rickettsii is the bacterium that causes RMSF, which is spread by the American dog tick. Fever, rash, headaches, and sore muscles are among the symptoms. If antibiotics are not taken quickly, RMSF can be lethal.

3. Ehrlichiosis:

Spread by the lone star tick, this illness is brought on by bacteria belonging to the Ehrlichia genus. Fever, chills, headache, and muscle aches are some of the symptoms. Severe cases may result in complications like breathing problems and renal failure.

4. Anaplasmosis:

Anaplasma phagocytophilum is the bacteria that causes anaplasmosis, which is spread by the blacklegged tick. Fever, headache, chills, and muscle aches are some of the symptoms. Severe consequences may arise if left untreated, particularly in those with compromised immune systems.

5. Babesiosis:

Spread by the blacklegged tick, babesiosis is caused by protozoan parasites of the genus *Babesia*. It damages red blood cells and, especially in those with weakened immune systems, can result in symptoms ranging from moderate flu-like symptoms to a serious, life-threatening sickness.

6. Alpha-gal Syndrome:

The bite of a lone star tick transfers a sugar molecule known as alpha-gal into the circulation, resulting in this unusual disease. This may set off an allergic reaction to red meat, resulting in symptoms including swelling, hives, and in more serious situations, anaphylaxis.

Preventive and Therapeutic Measures

Avoiding tick-borne illnesses requires preventing tick bites. Here are a few successful tactics:

1. Apply Insect Repellents:

Spray exposed skin and clothing with insect repellents that contain DEET, picaridin, or oil of lemon eucalyptus. Ticks are effectively repelled by these repellents.

2. Wear Protective Clothing:

Wear long sleeves, long pants, and closed-toe shoes if you're going to be in an area where ticks are common. To stop ticks from climbing up your legs, tuck your jeans into your socks. You can more quickly identify ticks if you wear light-colored clothing.

3. Treat Clothing and Gear:

Treat clothing, shoes, and camping gear with permethrin, an insecticide that kills ticks on contact. Pre-treated clothing is also available and provides long-lasting protection.

4. Avoid Tick Habitats:
Stay on well-maintained pathways and avoid going through tall grass, brush, and leaf litter where ticks are usually found.

5. Perform Tick Checks:
After spending time outdoors, thoroughly check your body, clothing, and pets for ticks. Pay particular attention to regions where ticks are prone to hide, such as underarms, groin, scalp, and behind the ears.

6. Remove Ticks Quickly:
Use fine-tipped tweezers to remove any ticks that are clinging to your skin as soon as

you discover them. Take hold of the tick as near the skin's surface as you can, then drag it upward with even, steady pressure. Use an antiseptic or soap and water to clean the bite area.

7. Keep an Eye Out for Symptoms: Following a tick bite, keep an eye out for signs of illnesses carried by ticks, such as fever, rash, exhaustion, and muscular aches. If you encounter any strange symptoms, get medical help, especially if you reside in or have been to a region where tick-borne illnesses are common.

Ticks are resilient, sophisticated parasites that have a big effect on people's health. Effective management and prevention depend on an understanding of the different species, their life cycles, and the distinctions between males and females. Ticks are becoming more common as a result of urbanization and climate change, thus prevention and awareness are essential. To lessen the likelihood of insect bites and the diseases they can spread, it's sensible to use repellents, wear protective clothes, and regularly check for ticks. We may better defend ourselves and our loved ones from these invasive pests by being aware of our surroundings and alert.

Chapter 2: A Comprehensive Guide

Ticks are little, hazardous arachnids that cling to human and animal skin in order to feed on blood. Although tick bites are generally not harmful, they can occasionally result in more serious conditions such anaplasmosis, Rocky Mountain spotted fever, and Lyme disease. To lower the risk of these illnesses, proper removal of ticks is essential. This document offers recommendations on what to do after removing ticks, along with step-by-step instructions for doing so safely.

Elimination Methods

It's critical to remove ticks promptly and accurately in order to stop the spread of disease. To remove ticks safely, use these instructions:

1. Set Up Your Equipment:
Assemble the required equipment prior to extracting the tick. You will need rubbing alcohol or soap and water, a small container (ideally with a cover) to store the tick for identification if necessary, and a pair of fine-tipped tweezers.

2. Clean the Area :
Use soap and water to give your hands a good wash. Use soap and water or rubbing alcohol to clean the region surrounding the

tick bite. This lowers the chance of contracting an infection.

3. Grasp the Tick with Tweezers:

Take hold of the tick as near the skin's surface as you can with tweezers that have fine tips. To avoid compressing the tick's body and causing it to discharge additional infectious material into your skin, avoid using your fingers to remove the tick.

4. Pull the Tick Out:

Lift the tick away from the skin by applying consistent, uniform pressure. The tick's mouthparts may break off and stay stuck in the skin if you twist or jerk the tick. Try using the tweezers to remove the mouthparts if they do break off. Leave them alone and allow the skin to heal if you are unable to remove them.

5. Get Rid of the Tick :

Put the tick in a little container and cover it. A plastic bag that is sealed will work also. To eliminate the tick, fill the jar with rubbing alcohol. Avoid using your fingers to crush the tick as this could expose you to any pathogens it may carry.

6. Clean the Bite Area Again:

Use soap and water or rubbing alcohol to thoroughly clean the bite area once the tick has been removed. This aids in avoiding any more infections.

7. Watch for Symptoms: For the next few weeks, keep a close check on the bite site. Keep an eye out for symptoms of infection, such as swelling, redness, or the emergence of a rash. Systemic symptoms such as fever, chills, exhaustion, aches in the muscles, or discomfort in the joints may be signs of a disease carried by ticks.

What to do after Removal

The procedure of removal itself is not as crucial as proper post-removal care. To make sure you stay healthy after having a tick removed, take the following actions:

1. Save the Tick for Identification:

Keep the tick in the container for identification if you reside in a region where tick-borne illnesses are prevalent. In the event that you exhibit symptoms of a tick-borne illness, this may prove beneficial to medical practitioners. Put the bite location and date on the container's label.

2. Watch for evidence of Infection:

It's important to keep an eye out for tick-borne illnesses or evidence of infection in the bite location after removing a tick. After the bite, symptoms may show up a few days to many weeks later. A bullseye-shaped rash, which is indicative of Lyme disease, or redness around the bite site are common warning signs to look out for:

- Fatigue, headache, cold, or muscle aches.

- Swollen lymph nodes in the vicinity of the bite.

3. Seek Medical Attention if Necessary:

Get in touch with your healthcare practitioner right away if you have any tick-borne illness symptoms. Tell them about the date of the tick bite, the bite itself, and any symptoms you are having. The prevention of severe sequelae from diseases carried by ticks is contingent upon early diagnosis and treatment.

4. Consider Preventive Antibiotics:

If the tick bite occurs in a region where Lyme disease is highly prevalent and if the tick has been attached for longer than 36 hours, your doctor may in certain circumstances advise a single dosage of antibiotics as a preventive step. This choice is influenced by various elements, including the kind of tick, when it attaches, and the frequency of tick-borne illnesses in the region.

5. Protect Your Pets:

Diseases carried by ticks can also affect pets. Once the tick has been removed from your pet, keep an eye out for any symptoms of sickness, including as lethargy, appetite loss, lameness, or swollen joints. Should your pet exhibit any symptoms, speak with your veterinarian. To keep your pets safe from tick bites, use the products your veterinarian has prescribed on a regular basis.

6. Avoid Future Tick Bites:

Take action to avoid getting bitten by ticks in the future. When strolling through places with grass or trees, wear long sleeves and pants. Make use of insect repellents containing picaridin, DEET, or oil of lemon eucalyptus. Use permethrin, an insecticide that kills ticks upon contact, on clothing and equipment. After spending time outside, regularly check for ticks on your family, yourself, and your pets.

7. Prevent Ticks in Your Yard:

Ticks prefer wet, shady areas with lots of leaf litter and tall grass. To prevent ticks from entering your yard, mow the lawn frequently and keep the grass short.

- Clearing the area surrounding your house of brush, long grasses, and leaf litter.

- Making a 3-foot-wide barrier out of gravel or wood chips between your lawn and any wooded areas to create a tick-safe zone.

- Carefully stacking wood in a dry location to deter rodents that may harbor ticks.

- Reducing tick populations in your yard by using items designed to control tick populations, like acaricides.

8. Educate Others and Yourself:

Learn about diseases carried by ticks and how to avoid them. Inform your loved ones, neighbors, and the community about the dangers posed by ticks and the significance of appropriately removing them. Engage in neighborhood initiatives to lower tick numbers and raise public knowledge of ticks.

Ticks can spread dangerous diseases to both humans and animals, making them more than simply a bother. To reduce the risk of illness, proper tick removal is crucial. You may prevent tick-borne infections for yourself and your loved ones by adhering to the step-by-step instructions for safe tick removal and taking the necessary precautions after removal. Recall to keep an eye out for symptoms, get help if needed, and take precautions to lessen the chance of getting bitten by a tick in the future. It is possible to enjoy the outdoors and avoid the risks associated with ticks by exercising caution and monitoring.

Chapter 3: Preventing Tick Bite Injury

Ticks are tiny but powerful disease-carrying insects that can afflict both people and animals. Despite being a natural component of many ecosystems, they can seriously endanger human health. Preventing tick bites and the diseases they carry is the best defense against tick bites for you and your family. To keep you safe, this book includes effective repellents and treatments, clothes and equipment for protection, yard upkeep, and tick control.

Effective Treatments and Repellents

It is essential to use the proper repellents and treatments to prevent tick infestation. The following are a few of the best choices:

1. DEET:

One of the most widely used and potent components in insect repellents is DEET (N, N-Diethyl-meta-toluamide). Tick protection lasting many hours can be achieved with products containing 20% to 30% DEET. Avoid getting repellant in your mouth, eyes, or open wounds; instead, apply it only to exposed skin and clothing.

2. Picaridin:

Picaridin is another extremely potent repellent that has a less greasy feel and a more attractive scent than DEET. It is frequently regarded as being just as effective as DEET. It offers enduring defense against ticks and is safe to apply to skin and clothing.

3. Oil of Lemon Eucalyptus:

Research has shown that oil of lemon eucalyptus (OLE), a natural substitute for synthetic chemicals, works well against ticks. Products with 30% OLE can offer defense for as long as six hours. Keep in mind that using OLE on children less than three is not advised.

4. Permethrin:

Applied to clothing and equipment instead of the skin, permethrin differs from DEET and picaridin. Ticks are repelled and killed upon contact by garments treated with permethrin; this action lasts for multiple washings. You can use permethrin spray to treat your own clothing or purchase already treated items.

5. Tick Repellent for Pets:

The diseases that ticks carry can also infect pets through tick bites. Use tick preventive products for your pets that have been advised by veterinarians, such as collars, spot treatments, or oral drugs. Check your pets for ticks on a regular basis, especially after they have been outside.

Protective Clothes and Equipment

When spending time in tick-prone locations, using the appropriate clothing and equipment can dramatically lower the chance of tick bites.

1. Long Sleeves and Pants:

Wear long sleeves and long pants if you're going on a hike or working in an area where ticks are common. To stop ticks from climbing up your legs, tuck your jeans into your socks. Ticks will find it more difficult to penetrate this barrier and get to your skin.

2. Light-Colored Clothes:

Light-colored clothes makes ticks easier to see. If you dress in white or light-colored clothing, it will be easier to spot ticks and remove them before they get attached to your skin.

3. Treated Clothing:

For further protection, put on permethrin-treated clothing. You have the option of treating your own clothes at home or buying pre-treated garments. A permethrin application adds an extra line of defense against ticks and endures through multiple washes.

4. Hats and Headgear:

Ticks can be deterred from attaching themselves to your scalp and hair by donning a hat. For added protection, think about donning headgear that has been permethrin-treated.

5. Boot Covers and Gaiters:

These items offer an additional degree of defense for your feet and lower limbs, which are frequently ticks' first points of contact. These are particularly helpful while moving through dense undergrowth or tall grass.

6. Insect Shield Products:

This brand sells a variety of apparel and equipment that has been permethrin-treated. Socks, caps, bandanas, and other items that can shield you from tick bites fall under this category.

Ticks can spread a number of diseases, which makes them a serious health risk. A variety of measures must be taken to prevent tick bites, such as using potent repellents, wearing protective clothes and equipment, maintaining a well-kept yard, and controlling tick populations. You may greatly lower your risk of tick bites and enjoy the outdoors with more peace of mind by using these equipment and suggestions.

Remain up to date on tick activity in your neighborhood, check yourself, your family, and your pets frequently, and remove ticks promptly if you discover any. The best defense against diseases carried by ticks is prevention, and you can protect your family and yourself from these invasive pests by putting the appropriate plans in place.

Conclusion

Ticks carry many dangerous diseases that can harm both humans and animals globally, making them more than simply a bother. The need for cutting edge research and creative preventative measures grows more pressing as tick populations and the diseases they transmit continue to expand.

Progress in the Knowledge of Tick-Borne Illnesses

1. Genomic Research on Pathogens and Ticks:
The genomes of ticks and the diseases they transmit have been sequenced by scientists thanks to recent developments in genomic

technologies. Understanding tick biology, behavior, and disease transmission processes requires knowledge of this genetic information. For example, scientists are utilizing genomic data to pinpoint the genes found in tick saliva, which comprises substances that aid ticks in avoiding host immunological reactions. Comprehending these mechanisms may facilitate the creation of vaccinations or therapies that specifically target these genes.

2. Research on the Microbiome:

Tick biology and disease transmission are significantly influenced by their microbiome, which is made up of bacteria, viruses, and other microbes. The ways in which these microorganisms interact with the tick host and each other are becoming clearer through research on the tick microbiome. It might be feasible to lessen ticks' capacity to spread infections by adjusting the microbiome. This strategy may result in novel biological control techniques that are sustainable and kind to the environment.

3. Pathogen Detection and Diagnostics: Molecular biology developments have produced extremely sensitive and targeted diagnostic instruments for the identification of pathogens carried by ticks. Pathogens at very low quantities can be quickly identified with methods like next-generation sequencing (NGS) and polymerase chain reaction (PCR). These instruments are essential for the early detection and management of diseases carried by ticks,

which may lessen the intensity and length of illnesses.

4. Immune Response Studies:

Another crucial field of study is how the immune system reacts to infections carried by ticks and tick bites. Research is being conducted to examine the immune responses in various hosts, including humans, in order to determine possible targets for vaccinations. For instance, scientists are investigating whether human immunity to tick bites might be developed through similar mechanisms in certain species.

5. Longitudinal Surveillance:

To monitor changes in tick populations and the occurrence of diseases carried by ticks, long-term surveillance studies are necessary.

These studies offer important information on the effects of environmental changes, such as urbanization and climate change, on tick dispersal and disease transmission. Predicting future epidemics and creating preventive public health initiatives require this information.

Novel Approaches to Tick Management

1. Vaccine Development:

Developing vaccinations is one of the most promising approaches to tick control. Vaccines that target ticks and the infections they carry are being developed by researchers. The goal of a tick vaccination would be to cause an immunological reaction in the host that would hinder the tick's capacity to feed or proliferate. Conversely, vaccines that target specific pathogens, like Lyme disease, would try to stop the sickness from spreading.

2. Genetic Engineering and CRISPR:

There is a lot of promise for tick control with the application of genetic engineering techniques like CRISPR. Researchers are looking into how to modify tick or pathogen genomes via CRISPR editing. Gene drives might be employed, for instance, to disseminate genes that decrease ticks' ability to reproduce or spread illness. Even though this technology is still in its infancy, it offers a promising path forward for tick control initiatives in the future.

3. Biological Control Agents:

Using diseases, parasites, or natural predators to manage tick populations is known as biological control. For example, it has been discovered that some nematodes and fungi are efficient against ticks. Scholars are presently exploring methods to improve the effectiveness and durability of these biological control agents. Another tactic being investigated is the introduction or enhancement of natural predators, such as specific bird species or rodents that consume ticks.

4. Environmental Management:

Reducing tick habitats through environmental management is a doable and frequently quick solution to tick control. Techniques include changing the environment to discourage wildlife, especially deer, from entering residential areas by removing bushes and tall grasses, which are breeding grounds for ticks. Taking these precautions can greatly lower the chance of coming into contact with ticks.

5. Integrated Pest Management (IPM):
IPM successfully manages tick populations by combining a number of control techniques. This strategy combines biological controls, environmental management, public education, and chemical controls like acaricides. The objective is to minimize the usage of hazardous chemicals while utilizing a combination of economically and environmentally sound techniques.

6. Wearable Technologies and Smart Fabrics:

Novel approaches to preventing tick bites are provided by advancements in wearable technology and smart fabrics. Tick-detection fabrics and apparel sprayed with persistent repellents are being developed by researchers. An early warning system and a decreased chance of tick bites can be achieved by integrating smart fabrics with sensors that notify the wearer when a tick is detected.

7. Public Health Campaigns and Education:

Two essential elements of tick control are education and public awareness. Successful public health campaigns can inform the public about the dangers of diseases carried by ticks and the precautions they can take to stay safe. This contains details on how to remove ticks properly, how to apply repellents, and how important it is to regularly check for ticks after being outside.

8. Smart Surveillance Systems:

The creation of smart surveillance systems to monitor disease outbreaks and tick populations is made possible by technological advancements. These systems forecast and track tick activity in real time by using machine learning techniques, remote sensing, and geographic information systems (GIS). By using this data, public health initiatives can be better targeted in halting the spread of diseases carried by ticks.

Since tick-borne illnesses are still a major threat to the public's health, it is imperative that research and innovation continue in order to provide preventative and control measures that work. Research on pathogen detection, microbiome, genomics, immune response, and pathogen detection is improving our knowledge of tick biology and disease transmission.

Promising approaches to managing tick populations and lowering the risk of tick-borne diseases include vaccine development, genetic engineering, biological control agents, environmental management, and integrated pest management.

Smart surveillance systems, wearable technology, and public health initiatives are all crucial elements of a thorough tick control plan. We can strengthen our ability to defend ourselves and our communities against the threats posed by ticks and the diseases they carry by combining these strategies and keeping up our investments in research and innovation. Tick-borne disease's potential to drastically lower global public health impacts makes the future of tick research and prevention bright.